WEIGHT LOSS FOR VEGANS

The Only Guide You Will Ever Need

Charles Thornton

DEDICATION

This is dedicated to people who want results.

CONTENTS

Introduction

Weight loss plans fail. It's a fact. Why then are we so confident that this one will help? Several reasons.

First, let's look at why most weight loss plans fail miserably.

There's one reason behind them, but the reason is so important it is the grave of many diets.

The reason is deprivation. Most weight loss plans call for it, and for no good reason, too. According to the average weight loss plan out there, you have to have patience and survive these first few weeks, valiantly battling cravings, eating less than you ever did in your life, and struggling to find the flavor of the bland dishes prescribed.

You manage. You pull through. You complete the weight loss plan, and go back to your old life, only to put that weight back on.

Deprivation-based weight loss plans simply don't work. You can't deprive yourself for your entire life. What you can do is change some of the habits that make you put on the weight. You won't have to cavalry-charge them like a fairy-tale knight too. And you won't have to perform feats of patience of willpower. All you have to do is want to improve. Gradually. Without heroics. Slow and steady wins the race. Slow and steady loses weight.

This short book is going to explain the theory and practice behind weight loss, and it's geared specifically towards vegans. It deals with weight loss, but it also takes into account pros and cons of a vegan diet. It describes minerals and vitamins vegans are most likely to be deficient in when dieting, and it explains how to get enough essential nutrients to feel better than ever while losing weight the vegan way.

If you are anxious to start right now, start with the part called "The

Practice".

It describes the steps that you need to take to start your final weight loss journey.

Be sure to take your time and learn The Theory too. You will understand why you are doing what you are doing, and it is going to let you expand your options and motivate you on your quest.

Let's begin.

.

THE THEORY

When we speak about weight loss, what words come to mind? For some its Atkins diet, low-fat diet or maybe color-diet. For others, exercise comes to mind, be it cardio or resistance training, cycling or swimming, working out in the gym or jogging. Most people will give both answers. Most people will say that in order to lose weight, a combination of exercise and diet is in order.

What is so magical about this diet-exercise pair that makes everyone think of it when the weight loss topic comes up? Well, to put it bluntly, that's because it works. Diet and exercise will help anyone lose weight, no exception.

Why, then, many people report that dieting or exercise doesn't work, and why so many struggle with losing their weight? After all, everyone knows that if you just exercise and go on a diet, you will get slimmer, fitter, happier, healthier, the list of benefits are endless. Why then for so many this formula just doesn't work, especially with all the information out there that helps people pick ideal weight loss plans for them?

Well, in addition to the reason stated in the introduction, there's just too much information.

You don't have to know a lot to lose weight. You certainly don't have to know about tons of existing diets that claim to help you lose weight. What you need to know are the core concepts behind weight loss, the most important of which is the Calories In, Calories Out principle.

Calories In, Calories Out

You've probably heard about this. If you did some research, odds are you know that there are conflicting opinions on the calories in, calories out principle. For the sake of readers who see this formula for the first time, and for the sake of clarity, let's recap on this a bit.

Calories In, Calories Out (CICO) is basically a model of how our bodies deal with calories. The goal of the model is to simplify its real-life representation to make it easier to understand and study, and the Calories In, Calories Out model does just that.

The model views human body as something like a car, and calories as fuel. Calories from food go in, the body can go a certain distance, or perform other activities. If calories from food provide more energy than needed for the activities performed, weight is gained in form of fat. If calories from food provide less energy, weight is lost.

Calories In – Calories Out = Weight Loss.

That's the gist of it. Since it's a model, it's inherently an oversimplification. For that reason, it's been receiving a lot of undeserved flak recently. Let's look it over in more detail to understand it better.

Calories In

A dietary calorie, AKA kilogram calorie or kcal, is the measure of energy required to heat one kilogram of water by one degree Celsius.

If you take a hamburger worth 400kcal and completely burn it, it will heat a kilogram of water by 400 degrees Celsius. Amazing, right? That's actually almost how the caloric content of foods is determined. Almost. Most foods have indigestible substances, like fiber, in them. And while they burn well and good, they can't be digested by our bodies. Simply burning a whole hamburger doesn't provide an accurate estimate of how much energy will human body derive from food, since fiber, which can't be digested, will still be counted towards the total energy of the food.

That's why a method known as Atwater system is used. The method involves simply adding up the calories available from the nutrients, which can be digested, of the food item. The calories available from the nutrients are determined just by burning them separately, and measuring the water temperature.

Here's the list of these nutrients, and the associated caloric values:

- **Carbohydrates** (this includes sugars and starches, with your basic table sugar or honey being the prime example) contain 4kcal per gram.
- **Proteins** (the building blocks of your body which are very important, rarely encountered in their pure form) contain 4kcal per gram.
- **Fats** (butter, olive oil, and so on) contain 9kcal per gram.
- **Ethanol** (beer, wine, spirits) contain 7kcal per gram.

Now, remember the method by which the caloric content of these nutrients was determined? That's right, they were simply burned down. And while all of them are digestible, and the first law of thermodynamics states that this energy has to go somewhere – it can't just disappear – it doesn't mean that eating 500kcal worth of food means the same thing for everyone. In fact, it doesn't even mean the same thing when we look at different nutrients as source of calories.

This brings us to two very important conclusions:

1. People are not bomb calorimeters (the devices used to measure the caloric content). While all people use energy

derived from food in the same way, the efficiency by which they convert food into energy varies. No two people get the same amount of usable energy from the same 500kcal hamburger. However, not a single person can derive more than 500kcal from a 500kcal food. Only less. What this means is, when you look at the nutritional profile of food, it gives you the maximum energy you can derive from it, no matter your metabolism, making it possible for everyone to lose weight by eating less.

2. While a calorie is just a calorie, people, again, are not calorimeters. The source of the calories matters. For the purpose of weight loss or gain, it's important to remember that while an average human being can get almost all of the energy from fats and carbohydrates, they get utilized differently. We will get into the details of which sources of energy are preferable for weight loss in the next chapters.

The bottom line: It's impossible to get more calories from the food than stated on the label, no matter the metabolism, so the Calories In principle is correct. However, it's important to remember that calorie is not just a calorie. Our bodies treat calories received from different sources differently. That's why gorging on sweets, which are essentially sugar and fat combined, is counterproductive to weight loss, even if you meet your calories in quota.

Calories Out

At this point, some of you might be thinking, "Wait. Now just what does this have to do with dieting? What does it matter if some water somewhere is heated?" The connection is actually rather simple. When we consume a calorie worth of food, we essentially eat energy (sounds pretty New Age-y, right?). And according to the first law of thermodynamics, that energy cannot disappear or be destroyed. It can only change form, or be used in some way.

What happens to that energy that we consume in form of food?

Well, since our temperature doesn't increase every time we eat a cookie, it doesn't just heat the water inside us, right? So what does it do?

Well, most of the energy goes towards letting us stay alive.

We need energy just to keep our heart, lungs, liver, intestines, the nervous system, including the brain, working properly. The amount of energy required for our body just to stay alive is called **basal metabolic rate, or BMR.** The bulk of calories spent by an average human goes towards meeting the basal metabolic rate. The BMR is not fixed. It depends on many factors, which include age, gender, muscle mass, and so on. Fortunately, it's easy to calculate. In fact, why don't you do that right now?

Here are the formulas, different for men and women:

Men BMR = 88.362 + (13.397 x weight in kg) + (4.799 x height in cm) - (5.677 x age in years)

Women BMR = 447.593 + (9.247 x weight in kg) + (3.098 x height in cm) - (4.330 x age in years)

Let's say Joe is 25 years old, 180cm tall, and weighs 70kgs. His basal metabolic rate would be:

88.362 + (13.397 x 70kg) + (4.799 x 180cm) – (5.677 x 25 years) = 1748kcal.

That's how much energy he needs each day just to stay alive. Now calculate your own BMR.

Then comes the question of activity. That's the "exercise" component of a weight loss program. How can you add that? Well, you have two options. You either find how many calories does a specific activity burn or you multiply your BMR by a number that corresponds to your activity level. Considering the differences in intensity, how different people expend energy, and other factors, attempting to calculate caloric expenditure for each and every activity often ends up being as much of an approximation as multiplying the BMR by a number corresponding to the activity level. Still, both ways create a good starting point which gives you a general idea of where your diet is headed.

Little to no exercise	Daily kilocalories needed = BMR x 1.2
Light exercise (1–3 days per week)	Daily kilocalories needed = BMR x 1.375
Moderate exercise (3–5 days per week)	Daily kilocalories needed = BMR x 1.55
Heavy exercise (6–7 days per week)	Daily kilocalories needed = BMR x 1.725
Very heavy exercise (twice per day, extra heavy workouts)	Daily kilocalories needed = BMR x 1.9

If our Joe exercises regularly, and his activities invariably end up in him sweating and panting, having difficulties speaking, then we can conclude he is doing heavy exercise, and multiply his BMR of 1748kcal by 1.725.

1748kcal x 1.725=3015kcal.

3015kcal is how much energy he has to get from food to keep his bodyweight stable.

The bottom line: Calories In, Calories Out model is sound, and it works. While it is not supposed to provide an absolutely accurate result of the number of calories consumed and spent, it gives a good estimation of how much calories one spends. This number is calculated using the following formula for the appropriate gender:

Men BMR = 88.362 + (13.397 x weight in kg) + (4.799 x height in cm) - (5.677 x age in years)

Women BMR = 447.593 + (9.247 x weight in kg) + (3.098 x height in cm) - (4.330 x age in years)

And then applying the changes needed to represent the level of activity of the person in question.

Calculating Fat Loss Using Calories In Calories Out

By now we've established that the CICO model is, while by no means absolutely accurate, can be used to provide an estimate of how many calories a person consumes, and how many calories a person expends.

How does all of this relate to fat loss?

Simple. Just put the daily calories value into the CICO equation. For our Joe, the number is 3015kcal, so the whole thing looks like this:

Calories In – 3015kcal = caloric balance.

Now, if caloric balance is negative, meaning Calories In are less than Calories Out, or 3015kcal in the case of Joe, weight loss happens.

Let's say Joe is eating 2515kcal a day. Then the formula looks like this:

2515kcal – 3015kcal = -500kcal.

Joe can't get these 500kcal out of thin air. He doesn't get them from food. Where does he get them? From his fat. As stated earlier, the caloric value of 1 gram of fat is 9kcal. This means that a person with a 100% efficient metabolism is able to get 9000kcal out of a kilogram of fat, or 3500kcal out of a pound of fat. Metabolism of most people is not as efficient, and they actually get a bit less calories from fat, but for the sake of weight loss, using 3500kcal a pound is good enough.

Now, if our Joe keeps his caloric deficit of 500kcal up for a week, he is going to lose a pound of fat by the weekend.

Let's recap

Calories In, Calories Out principle works. There's no doubt about it. Of course, all people are different. For some, metabolism is more efficient. Others are less efficient at converting food to energy. However, it's impossible to get more calories out of a food that it is stated on a label. It's also impossible to get more calories than 3500 out of a pound of fat.

That's why the Calories In part works.

On the other hand, the Basal Metabolic Rate and the daily caloric requirement can be very different for many people. Unfortunately, there is no way to find out your exact Basal Metabolic Rate. The only thing you can do is calculate the approximate BMR and work from there, using the trial and error method.

One other thing that is important to remember is that if you want to sustainably lose fat, minimizing your caloric intake drastically is a very, very bad idea. First of all, it's one of the unhealthiest things one can do in relation to the diet. Secondly, it is counterproductive on the long run, as when caloric intake is too low, the body will start to cannibalize muscle tissue along with fat, which both decreases the BMR and invariably leads to certain health issues. If you have a friend who starved themselves for a week, lost weight, and was just fine, it doesn't mean the starvation didn't cost them health. It's just the effect is not obvious immediately.

Beyond the Calories

As we already established, calorie is not just a calorie. The success of your weight loss effort does not depend on just the caloric deficit. It also depends on the specific foods you eat, or don't eat.

And while vegans are safe from many bad food choices just by choosing to lead a vegan lifestyle, there are many things that still should be left behind in order to sustainably lose weight.

First, let's talk about the specific macro- and micronutrients.

Macronutrients

What is a macronutrient and which functions do they perform in the body? Let's start with the definition.

Macronutrients are substances that our bodies require in large amounts in order to grow and function properly. Macronutrients are your main source of calories, and the only thing besides alcohol that plays the role in the Calories In part of the equation. They include fats, carbohydrates, and protein. Alcohol isn't considered a macronutrient because we do not need it for survival, or to function properly, at least as far as the physiological point of view is concerned.

Let's take a closer look at each of the macronutrients.

Protein

Proteins are organic molecules, which are made up of amino acids. Proteins are found in abundance in foods such as meat, dairy, or beans. In a vegan diet, the most important sources of proteins are beans, legumes, and nuts. Grains, fruits, and vegetables usually have low protein content. Protein is the most important macronutrient in anyone's diet, and here's why.

Proteins are actually large chains which consist of molecules known as amino-acids. You've probably heard of them. Odds are, you also have heard they are very important for the proper function of human body, and that essential and non-essential amino-acids exist. Amino acids are what makes your body work properly. They are needed both to support and build muscle – all muscle, which includes not only biceps, but your heart and lungs – and to help carry out many, many chemical reactions of your body.

For instance, tyrosine amino acid causes you to feel alert and active, while also controlling your thyroid gland. Low levels of tyrosine equal low activity of thyroid gland, and this in turn impacts weight-loss. In fact, tyrosine deficiency can potentially create a vicious circle. If a person has a diet low in tyrosine, obesity due to low activity of thyroid can take place. As the person struggles to eat less, they receive even less dietary tyrosine, which only serves to exacerbate the problem. And that's just one amino acid. The same can happen when an overweight person attempts to lose weight by simply cutting their caloric intake, without actually looking at which foods they eat. If there are not enough amino acids in the diet, thyroid problems are only one potential problem that can arise.

In fact, here are the symptoms that you are not getting enough protein in your diet:

1. Lack of energy or motivation. This is self-explanatory. You have less energy than before, you feel sleepy and tired all the time, and you start losing the will to live. Most often than not, the cause is lack of protein.
2. You become weaker. Your muscles require a constant flow of protein to repair them. This is especially true for anyone doing any sports, but those living a sedentary lifestyle can experience this, too. If you are not getting enough protein, your muscles can't repair themselves when the protein that constitutes them degrades, and over time, you lose strength.

3. You actually lose visible muscle. This marks a serious issue with your diet. Your body needs protein to support all kinds of chemical reactions to stay healthy and survive. When you don't get enough protein with food, guess what? Your body is going to start eating away at your own muscles just to stay alive, with potentially dire consequences. You won't only be losing muscle mass and strength. You will also end up with a wide array of conditions, as after all, your heart and lungs are muscles too.

4. Your nails become brittle, your hair could start falling out, and your wounds don't heal as quickly. This is another alarming symptom of protein deficiency. If your wounds, even superficial ones such as scratches, are not healing as quickly as they used to, and if you are noticing more hair on your pillow than usual, then it's time to increase your protein intake.

These symptoms are just some of the most noticeable reasons why getting all the amino acids needed by the body is incredibly important both for weight loss and healthy living. And while there are many plant products that are rich in protein – peanuts come to mind – not all of them have all the amino acids needed for healthy functioning. This is because the proteins of certain foods, peanuts in our example, do not have the complete set of amino acids.

Fortunately, humans are remarkably resilient in many ways. Out of twenty-two amino acids that are significant for humans, we can synthesize about a dozen. The ten amino acids that we can't synthesize, however, have to be taken in from external sources. The essential amino acids are: Phenylalanine, Valine, Tryptophan, Threonine, Isoleucine, Methionine, Histidine, Arginine, Leucine, and Lysine. The list can be memorized using a mnemonic "Pvt. Tim Hall", if you want to appear smart and spoil everyone's appetite and mood during a meal.

Memorizing the list of these amino acids is not necessary. You don't have to check the make-up of each and every food to see if it has all the necessary amino acids. Most of the time, you will be getting them with every meal. It's just that some foods don't have that much of a certain amino acid.

For many vegans, this can be an issue. If there isn't much variety of protein sources, then it's easy to end up almost-deficient in a certain essential amino-acid. And while most of the times the effects are not very pronounced, over a long period this can develop into a full-blown deficiency and result in all kinds of unpleasantries. This is especially true for people who attempt to lose weight by cutting out calorie-dense foods, and the issue is especially sharp for dieting vegans, who may decide to cut things like beans, peas, nuts, or soy from their diet, instead subsisting on fruit, vegetables, and some grains.

Do not make this mistake, as that will undermine both your weight-loss effort and health. Instead, either stick to foods that have complete forms of protein in them, meaning proteins that have enough of essential and non-essential amino acids, or vary your protein sources with each meal.

A good rule of thumb is to eat both legumes and grains. Both of them are deficient in several essential amino-acids, but when consumed together, they complement each other, and you end up with a semblance of complete protein in your diet. This solution is far from ideal, but is definitely better than nothing, and one can probably live a healthy life of beans and grains. If the vegan in question participates in sports, however, a better source of protein is needed. Many people bash vegan diets claiming one cannot get good-quality protein on them. Nothing could be further from the truth.

Two of the best sources of complete protein available out there are completely, 100% vegan. Try to guess which.

If you said "soy", you've got half the answer. Soy is, simply put, a great nutritional choice. And while there are some things that have to be taken into account with it, it's still a real super food, densely packed with complete protein, all the amino acids your body needs (a bit low in Methionine, but not low enough for it to be significant), and minerals and vitamins such as copper, potassium, zinc, K, B9, B2, phosphorus, and more.

After soy, however, most folks are hard pressed to find the second half of answer. Yet it's one of the foods that is so common, popular, and traditional that we just fail to see the true value of it. It's easy to call something exotic a super food, but the reality is, yellow peas are an even better source of complete protein than soy. Yep, the modest yellow dry pea is a super food on par with soy, and in fact, even better than it. It has all the protein you can ever want, and is rich in many vitamins and minerals.

Finally, we have quinoa. While it almost made the list in that it is choke-full of vitamins and minerals, and can boast complete protein, it is not very high in it, and can be quite calorie-dense, which is an issue for a vegan trying to lose weight. 100g of raw quinoa have 14g of protein and 368kcal, while yellow peas have the same amount of calories – 364kcal per 100g – but with 21g of protein instead of 14. Soy, of course, takes the cake here, with 50g of protein and 346kcal per 100g.

What this basically means is that any vegan should include two of three sources of protein in their diets to ensure that they are getting enough essential amino acids:

Soy
Yellow peas
Quinoa

This list is very simplified, and by looking at specific nutritional profiles of various foods, any of these foods can be substituted by other choices. Still, there is no reason to ignore obviously healthy foodstuffs, and while soy receives a lot of bad rep because of its high phytoestrogen content, research shows that unless one is eating several kilograms of soy a day, it's absolutely safe.

Speaking of several kilograms – just how much protein a day should a healthy person take in?

The answer largely relies on the type and intensity of your activities. As you know, the amino acids in protein are used both to sustain the chemical processes in the body, and to rebuild muscle. An average adult person should take in approximately 0.8g of protein per 1kg of bodyweight. Some weighing 70kg will be just fine if he's getting 50g of protein a day from varied sources, such as grains, legumes, and nuts.

The picture changes drastically when we are speaking about a growing child or someone who participates in heavy physical activity. In those cases, protein intake should be significantly higher, being within range of 1.5-2g of protein per 1kg of body weight a day. This number is dictated by a simple reason that in order to grow muscle, the body needs additional protein. 0.8g per 1kg is enough to sustain existing muscle. In case of a growing child, additional protein is needed so the body has enough materials to grow. In case of someone doing heavy physical activity, the picture is a bit different, as in certain cases, for instance when lifting a very, very heavy barbell, the muscles actually break down. Once the activity is over, the body attempts to rebuild the muscle, plus pack on some more, just in case. If there is not enough protein, the muscles will either be rebuilt to their original capacity, or in some cases, not recover completely, which over time will lead to loss of muscle mass, not a healthy thing.

There is one more thing to know about protein. While it's a very important macronutrient, and most of the times, the more you have of it, the better, it has two issues.

First, for someone with a pre-existing kidney condition, it can exacerbate it. Those with healthy kidneys need not worry, as consuming even 2g of protein per 1kg of body weight will not result in any health issues.

Second, protein is a building block of life. It's not a good source of fuel. This is both good and bad. For those trying to lose weight, protein is great because it spends a lot of time in the stomach and intestines. It's hard to break down, so it keeps people feeling full for a long period of time, as well as requiring a lot of energy to digest. It's estimated that 30% or so of the caloric value of protein is actually spent digesting it. Combine these two things, and you end up with a nutrient that keeps you sated for a long time and takes energy to digest.

The bad part is you can't have a diet based on protein as a source of fuel. The capacity of the human body to digest protein is limited, with the upper limit being approximately 350g of protein. When you consume over 350g of protein, you cannot digest it properly. This in return results in not having enough calories to maintain the energy balance, and in a variety of unpleasant symptoms such as diarrhea, low blood pressure and headache. What this means is that while a diet based only on protein may seem like a good weight loss option, other sources of energy are necessary for the proper functioning of the body.

The bottom line:

Protein is absolutely necessary for human survival. It regulates processes in the human body, including those in the brain, and serves as the body's building block. It's also a great weight loss macronutrient, since it keeps you sated for a long time and requires 30% of its caloric value to digest. However, one must ensure that one has an adequate intake of complete protein by including soy, yellow beans and quinoa in the diet, and making sure that at least 0.8g per 1kg of body weight is consumed daily.

Fat

Fats are the most calorie-dense type of macronutrient out there. One gram of fat has nine dietary calories, more than double the amount of proteins or carbohydrates. Fats also have the lowest "fullness" factor, meaning that people can eat more fat than protein or carbohydrate and still feel hungry. These two factors combined make fats one of the biggest culprits behind obesity and being overweight.

The problem is further exacerbated by the fact that many people over-consume saturated and trans-fats, which raise LDL, or "bad", cholesterol, and under-consume polyunsaturated fats, which are needed by the body both to lower LDL and increase HDL, or "good", cholesterol, and to serve a variety of other functions. In particular, some polyunsaturated fats are needed by the body to maintain cell membranes of most of the cells in the body, and to make prostaglandins, compounds which regulate various bodily processes.

The situation is pretty much the same as with proteins. Our bodies are able to synthesize most of the fatty acids needed for proper function. Still, there are some fatty acids which must be taken in from the outside, in the form of dietary fat. Fortunately, it's easy for vegans to get an adequate level of the so-called "essential" fatty acids. Even better, vegan diets are free from things like dietary cholesterol.

The three essential fatty acids that must be taken in from the dietary sources are all polyunsaturated. These are the only fats that you really need in your diet; the body can synthesize all others. Still, it's never a good idea to abruptly change the diet. If you were big on fats in your diet before, lower the intake gradually, until only polyunsaturated fats remain.

The three polyunsaturated fats that cannot be synthesized by the body and must be taken in with food or supplements are the Linoleic acid, Arachidonic acid, and Linonelinc acid; note that γ-linolenic acid is not essential, and is in fact very different from Linolenic acid. Don't confuse the two, as supplements and foods high in γ-linolenic acid won't do that much for your health.

Most vegans don't have to worry about the adequate supply of most essential fatty acids, since plant foods are the main source of them. However, those that choose to lose weight and subject themselves to extremely low-fat diets may show symptoms of essential fatty acid deficiency.

The symptoms include:

Allergic skin reactions, such as rash and eczema;
Other allergic reactions, such as asthma and hay fever;
Issues with vision, such as poor night vision, sensitivity to bright lights or difficulty reading;
Issues with attention, such as inability to concentrate, distractibility, and problems with working memory;
Emotional problems, including depression, mood swings, and anxiety;
Sleep problems, such as problems waking up in the morning or falling asleep at night;

Any of these symptoms signal a fatty acid deficiency. The chief vegan sources of essential fatty acids are the following:

Grape seed oil
Flax seed oil
Sunflower oil
Walnuts
Sunflower seeds
Full-fat soybeans
Pecan nuts
Peanuts

Even supplements are not necessary, however, since most of the nuts, as well as peanuts, include a generous amount of essential fatty acids. Still, nuts should be consumed in moderation due to their high fat content. Even a small serving of nuts can have a lot of calories, which can be an issue for people on a weight loss quest.

The bottom line:

Fatty foods are not a good choice for people trying to lose weight. The reasons behind it are that fat is very high in calories, two times more calorie dense than carbohydrates and proteins at 9 kcal per 1 gram, and doesn't provide a feeling of satiety. Still, cutting out all fats is bad, even when one is trying to lose weight, as human body depends on a dietary intake of three polyunsaturated fats: Linoleic acid, Arachidonic acid, and Linonelinc acid, the absence of which in the diet can cause health issues and unpleasant symptoms. For these reasons, sources of these essential fatty acids must be included in all diets, either in the form of supplement (grape seed oil, sunflower oil, flax seed oil), or from whole foods (nuts and beans).

Carbohydrates

Carbohydrates are the chief sources of energy that fuel the human body. By themselves, carbohydrates aren't essential nutrients. The human body can work without them just fine. That said, carbohydrate-rich foods often serve as sources of other more important nutrients such as fiber, vitamins and minerals, and completely cutting out carbohydrates from diet will cause a transitional phase when the body adapts to use fat as is its chief source of energy.

Carbohydrates can only be consumed by the human body in the form of monosaccharides.

There are two primary types of carbohydrates: "complex" and "simple" ones. The difference between the two is in the construction of their molecules. Simple carbohydrates are composed of mono- or disaccharides, while complex carbs are constructed of three or more molecules of sugar.

Very often, "simple" carbs are touted as bad, while "complex" carbs are considered good. Dividing sources of carbohydrates into foods containing "simple" or "complex carbs is not a good idea, however. The definitions of "simple" and "complex" carbs simply does not do the difference between them justice, especially when used in relation to weight loss. For instance, fruits and vegetables contain a lot of simple monosaccharides, which put them into the category of bad simple carbohydrates. On the other hand, whole grain bread, which can have a low amount of actual whole grain, with the bulk of it consisting of sugar and refined grain, is considered a complex carbohydrate, and is thus supposed to be better and more healthy than fruits and vegetables. In relation to weight loss, the whole thing is very misleading.

A more functional way to differentiate between carbohydrates is based on the way ingested foods are metabolized. Foods that cause a sharp rise in blood glucose and blood insulin contain functionally simple carbohydrates. Foods that cause a slow rise in blood glucose and insulin, on the other hand, should be considered to be a source of complex carbohydrates.

This notion of defining carbohydrates as being either simple or complex leads us to two very important concepts of Glycemic Index and Glycemic Load. Both are often spoken of, and sometimes are even interchanged. It's important to know the difference between the concepts of Glycemic Index and Glycemic Load. They are two different things which can make or break your diet.

Glycemic Index, or GI, shows how quickly the food is broken down into sugar in the bloodstream. Food with a higher GI raises blood sugar more quickly than food with lower GI. GI is very impractical when applied to dieting. According to GI, foods like carrots (GI of 47) cause a bigger increase in blood sugar than, say, spaghetti (GI of 44). Someone who depends on GI to tell if a certain food is suitable for a diet is bound to make a lot of mistakes using GI, since even common sense tells us that it's much easier to get lean on carrots than on spaghetti. This is because GI does not take into account the actual impact of the food on blood sugar. It only shows how fast the carbohydrates in the food are digested, and when to expect the effect to kick in.

Glycemic Load, on the other hand, provides a far more accurate measure of how carbohydrates from the food impact blood sugar. Glycemic Load, or GL, shows how much the blood sugar levels will actually rise. GL and GI of a single food can differ drastically. Let's look at carrots again. We already know that carrots have GI of 47. This shows that there are carbohydrates present in carrots that can be quickly absorbed. GL of carrots, on the other hand, is equal to just 4. That's because there are not much of the quick-absorbing carbohydrates in your average carrot. In the end, the impact of the food on the blood glucose level is better measured by Glycemic Load. Glycemic Index is still useful in certain cases, but it has to be used in conjunction with Glycemic Load to determine the actual impact the carbohydrate will have on blood levels.

Why is this important in the first place?

It's important because of the way human body deals with carbohydrates. When carbohydrates are ingested, they are broken down into monosaccharides in order to be absorbed. The process begins in the mouth with the release of saliva, and continues in stomach and intestines. As carbohydrates are broken down into monosaccharides and are absorbed, glucose from monosaccharides enters the blood stream. In healthy people, glucose from blood stream is transported to liver and muscles in order to replenish glycogen stores, which are depleted during activity. Glycogen is the substance which fuels human muscles. It's stored both in the muscle cells themselves and in the liver.

When a muscle performs work, it uses up glycogen, and if there is no glycogen available in the given muscle, glucose is taken up from the blood stream and is turned into glycogen. If there is not enough glucose present in the bloodstream, glycogen is taken up from the liver. If there is no glycogen in the liver, fat is broken down to provide fuel for the body.

If muscles and liver have enough glycogen, and foods with high Glycemic Load, such as candies, are consumed, the glucose still enters the bloodstream, but this time, the body turns it into fat instead of shuttling it to the muscle cells and the liver.

The reason why knowing about Glycemic Load of foods is important is because it's a good way to control how your body stores and burns its fat deposits. An average 70kg adult can store approximately 300g of glycogen at a given time. So for example if the adult in question performed an activity that took 1200 kcal of energy to perform, his glycogen stores would be depleted. After the glycogen stores are depleted, the body starts to use fat for energy.

On the other hand, if an adult with full glycogen storage consumes carbohydrates, they might or might not be turned into fat. This largely depends on the GI and GL of the food in question. If the GI and GL of carbohydrate consumed are low, then it will be digested and absorbed gradually. The glucose from the carbohydrate will enter the blood stream gradually as well, and the body can utilize it without turning it into fat to satisfy current energy needs.

If the food consumed is high both in GI and GL, it can be turned into fat even if the glycogen reserves are not full, simply because blood glucose levels spike too fast and too high for the body to efficiently utilize the glucose. This can partially refill glycogen stores and partially be turned into fat. Still, when low on glycogen – such as after a long session of exercise or any other activity that burned in excess of 1000 kcal – a high GI, healthy source of carbohydrates is a good option, as it helps the body not only to refill glycogen stores, but actually makes it store more glycogen, which will help next time one exercises.

As an energy source, carbohydrate is intermediate between fat and protein with regard to both energy density and satiety induction. Carbohydrate provides roughly 4 kcal per gram, which is generally considered to be just slightly more than that of protein. The satiety index of carbohydrate—meaning the degree to which a given "dose," measured in calories, induces a sense of fullness—is higher than that of fat and lower than that of protein. Complex carbohydrate is more satiating than simple carbohydrate, due largely to the fiber content. Fiber adds volume but not calories to food and soluble fiber may contribute to satiety by other mechanisms as well.

It's also worth noting that while most tissues accept glucose as well as other nutrients for fuel, brain and red blood cells can only use glucose. When there is not enough glucose for the brain to run on, the body breaks down fat in a special process known as ketosis. Ketosis is the principle behind low-carb diet and is claimed to provide faster fat loss than other types of diets. However, it's still subject to the Calories In – Calories Out principle, and is hard to implement on a vegan diet, as going low-carb may cause the vegan dieter to take in insufficient amount of nutrients from the diet.

The bottom line:
Carbohydrates are mostly used by the body as a fuel source and are remarkably efficient. Most people report feeling more

energetic on a high-carbohydrate diet as opposed to a high-fat diet. For vegans, a high-carbohydrate diet is more recommended than a high-fat diet, since it can be hard to get necessary nutrients, both micro and macro, while sacrificing carbs. One thing that's important to remember when trying to lose weight is to stick to foods with low GL. If both GI and GL are low, even better, but don't limit yourself to low GI foods only, as you will be missing out on a variety of healthy choices.

Micronutrients

Micronutrients are the stuff that our body needs is small amounts. Micronutrients include vitamins and minerals. There is a wide array of vitamins and minerals, but we are going to cover the specifics issues vegans might face in getting enough of their micronutrients daily.

This is because certain very important micronutrients are chiefly found in products of animal origin. There is no reason a vegan can't meet his micronutrient needs using only plant-based foods. The important thing here is keeping the menu as diverse as possible, while avoiding overly processed foods. However, many people may struggle with this, especially during a weight loss regimen, since many find it hard to cut down calories while keeping variety.

For this reason, a short list of micronutrients that vegans risk being deficient in, and of sources from which these micronutrients can be received, was compiled.

- **Iron**
  This micronutrient is important because it is a component of hemoglobin and myoglobin, two proteins involved in oxygen transportation, energy production and enzymatic functions.
  Symptoms of iron deficiency primarily include weakness and fatigue, and to a lesser degree difficulties concentrating and a weakened immune response.
  Foodstuffs such as apricots, raisins, prunes, peas, beans, spinach, and asparagus coupled with a citrus fruit are a good source of iron.
- **Zinc**

The mineral zinc is required for proper enzymatic functioning of protein synthesis, as well as immune function and wound healing.
Symptoms of zinc deficiency are loss of libido and sexual drive, decreased appetite, and slow wound healing.
Nuts are a good source of zinc.

- **Calcium**
Calcium is needed for bone health, as well as for muscle and neural activity.
Low intake of calcium means weakened bones, as well as loss of energy and strength.
Dark leafy green vegetables and also broccoli are great sources of calcium.

- **Vitamin D**
Vitamin D goes hand in hand with calcium, since vitamin D is required for the utilization of calcium during formation of bones.
Symptoms of vitamin D deficiency are the same as calcium deficiency.
Getting enough vitamin D is hard when maintaining a vegan diet and a supplement is recommended.

- **Vitamin B12**
Vitamin B12 is important for the same reason iron is important. B12 plays a role in the functioning of red blood cells, plus it is important for DNA formation.
Symptoms of vitamin B12 deficiency include anemia, fatigue, and neurological disorders.
Vitamin B12 should be supplemented when on a vegan diet, same as Vitamin D.

Why Junk Food is Junk

Our age is the age of junk foods. We have a lot of novel food choices, some of them, fake meat for example, aimed to make a life of vegan easier. In truth, they offer little to no nutritional benefit, and are obviously detrimental for any weight loss attempt.

The reason junk foods are bad is because they:

a) Contain a lot of calories
b) Contain little to no needed macronutrients
c) Contain little to no needed micronutrients
d) Often have a high GI and GL load

Basically, junk foods are just calories that go straight to fat. By now you already know that foods which are high in GI and GL are bad for you. They cause a rapid increase in blood sugar levels, which makes the human body utilize the excess of blood glucose as fat. This is the deal with junk food. Things like chocolate bars are so full of sugar that they invariably make the top of all GI and GL lists. As such, they cause a spike in blood sugar. The body is anxious to lower blood glucose, so only a part of consumed calories go towards replenishing glycogen stores. The other part is deposited into fat.

Furthermore, junk foods are very poor nutritional choices. They are usually cheap, and as such, every step is made to save money on the production process. For this reason, highly processed materials are used, materials which lack most of the micronutrients needed.

Finally, junk food is made to be superficially tasty, and humans are wired to like energy-dense, sweet and fatty things. Look at nutritional info of any junk food. You will see refined grains, sugars, and fats, plus a few additives to make the food more appealing. Basically what you end up with is a cup of sugar, a cup of oil, and a cup of flour, mixed together with some artificial aromas and colorings. You end up getting a lot of calories, but none of the protein or micronutrients that your body requires.

.

THE PRACTICE

If you didn't skip the theory part, kudos to you! You now know a whole lot more about the human body than you did before, you know how it functions, how it stores fat, how it loses fat, how to *make it* lose fat, the difference between macro and micronutrient, why GI and GL are important, and more.

For some, it might be too much to remember.

For others, it might be too long to read through.

Here's a short, quick, summary of the previous chapters, along with some new information. It describes what you are going to actually do to lose weight.

Oh. And remember, you can always look up nutritional profiles of specific foods using the http://nutritiondata.self.com/ website. There's no reason not to run every food you regularly eat through it. Do it.

Calories In

1) Counting calories

You will lose fat if you spend more calories than you consume. This is the fundamental of fundamentals. Abide by it, and you will lose fat. Fail to do so and your body won't change. Not a single diet will work, be it Atkinson, Paleo, or whatever else is out there, if you don't respect this principle. It works. It's practically a law of thermodynamics. Your body can't create energy out of thin air. Your body is, however, very efficient at turning food into energy. If the calories from food are not sufficient to fulfill your energy needs, the body will tap into its fat reserves, and use stored fat for energy. So to burn fat, you need to consume less calories. So **count your calories.**

How to count calories?

First, calculate your Basal Metabolic Rate (BMR) - the amount of calories your body needs just to perform basic functions like breathing, pumping blood, and generally not dying. Here's the formula:

Men BMR = 88.362 + (13.397 x weight in kg) + (4.799 x height in cm) - (5.677 x age in years)

Women BMR = 447.593 + (9.247 x weight in kg) + (3.098 x height in cm) - (4.330 x age in years)

Then, add your additional caloric needs to the BMR. Additional caloric needs are how much energy you burn during daily activities which are not related to breathing and other basic functions. Use the table provided in the Calories Out chapter.

The resulting number will probably end up being around 2000-2500 kcal a day, depending on your height, weight, gender, and activity level. Eat less than that, and you lose fat. Say your deficit is 500kcal a day. A pound of fat provides your body with 4500kcal, so every 9 days you're on a diet with a 500kcal deficit you will lose one pound of fat.

2) Don't starve yourself.

The optimal caloric deficit for fat loss is no more than 500kcal a day. This might seem counterintuitive, considering the previous principle. After all, if you don't eat at all, you will lose fat at a rapid rate, won't you? Frankly, you won't. One thing your body wants is to stay alive. If you stop eating at all, or have a caloric deficit of over 500kcal a day for a few days, your body will decide that something horrible is happening, and that food is scarce. If you starve yourself, your body will hold on onto its fat reserves for dear life, and instead will start breaking down muscles for energy, and lowering your Basal Metabolic Rate. Have a deficit of more than 500kcal a day, and you will lose muscle instead of fat, while feeling tired and lethargic.

The reason for this is very simple. Muscles require energy to maintain. The more muscle mass you have, the more energy you need to sustain them, in addition to supporting your basic life functions. When you starve yourself, your body decides that it's better to consume muscles for a double benefit of getting energy and decreasing future energy expenditure. Body fat, on the other hand, doesn't have any energy needs, so it's saved for later, as it costs nothing to maintain. This whole thing is called "starvation mode", and it saved the lives of many of our ancestors back before the Agricultural Revolution. Nowadays, however, it only sabotages the efforts of people who think it's better to eat nothing at all to lose fat faster.

3) Source of calories matters.

High-carbohydrate, high-protein, low-GI diets are best. What this means is, a diet high in vegetables, whole grains, yellow peas, soy, and stuff like that is better than a diet of, say, cookies and an occasional tomato, if there is a similar caloric deficit in both diets. There are several reasons behind this.

First, let's look at low GI. GI means Glycemic Index. To keep it very, very basic, foods with high GI are rapidly absorbed by your body, causing a spike of blood sugar. This blood sugar then quickly fulfills the energy needs of cells, then any excess blood sugar is rapidly turned into fat, and then you end up being a little bit fatter, and still hungry, because your blood sugar levels are low again. Foods with low GI index, on the other hand, are absorbed slowly, and steadily increase blood sugar by a small amount for a long period of time. This means that as your cells expend energy, they will steadily replenish it, but there won't be excess blood sugar, so you won't feel hungry, and won't gain fat.

Imagine eating 600kcal worth of chocolate (that's actually pretty close to a typical chocolate bar). It takes a few minutes to digest fully, and its full energy value has to be absorbed by the body. 600kcal is a lot, and your body doesn't really need that much energy at once. Your cells will replenish energy, taking, say, 300kcal, and the leftover 300 kcals get turned into fat. Half an hour later, when the cells expended some of the energy, you feel hungry again, because your blood sugar level is low. You give in to hunger and eat some more chocolate, gaining fat again, or you decide to stay hungry and feel weaker. That's an example of a high GI food.

Now imagine eating 600kcal of oatmeal. It takes a few hours to digest, so most of those 600kcal will go towards meeting the energy needs of your cells, with no additional fat gained. You don't feel hungry, and you don't gain fat. Win-win, and that's why low GI foods are great. You can look up GI values of various foods on the Internet.

The protein is similar to a low GI food in that it takes a long time to digest. It's also very important to your body, because it acts as a building block for skin, hair, muscle, internal organs, and also takes part in some important chemical processes. Finally, high carbohydrate means low fat, and this is great for your cardiovascular health.

Still, remember the first truth, no matter your diet, you need a caloric deficit to lose weight.

This is pretty much everything you need to know to lose weight effectively. Gaining muscle is a little bit trickier, because you will need a proper routine. You will also need to eat a lot of protein, and a good guideline for that is 0.8g of protein per 1kg of bodyweight.

To sum up:

1. Calculate your basal metabolic rate. Google how much calories a day your daily activity level requires. Add the two values. Substract 500. This is how much calories you should be eating a day to lose weight at a fastest rate possible without health problems.

2. Don't starve yourself. Having a deficit of more than 500kcal a day won't help you lose fat faster. It will hinder your fat loss efforts and make you lose muscles.

3. Eat a high-carbohydrate, high-protein, low-GI diet. No candies. No refined sugars. 50% of the calories comes from foods with a low GI and GL (the lower the better), 25-30% from protein, and the rest from fats. Very importantly, cut soda out. Many people can lose weight just by cutting out all soda from their diets.

Calories Out

Weight loss is primarily a result of diet. But guess what? A little physical activity goes a long way towards your health. Even if you don't play sports, consider dedicating just 20 minutes every other day to the workout proposed. You'll be grateful you did, as that will allow you to eat a bit more, and to feel a whole lot better. Plus you don't need anything but 20 minutes of your time for this one. No gym membership, no buying a bicycle, you don't even have to go outside to do this. Just make sure you warm up properly, and don't slack off. The results will come sooner than you expect.

Warm up
One very important thing to remember here is to keep the impact as low as possible. Imagine you are a ninja. Try to be as silent as you can; this makes you control your movement more, decreasing the impact and keeping your knees healthy.

1.   Start by **marching in place**, raising the knees up high when you march. A bit higher than your waist is ideal. Start out slow, gradually building up the pace.   Ten seconds slow, ten seconds moderate, and ten seconds full throttle.
2.   **Run in place.** Two tips here: your shins have to be parallel, and you should roll through the ball of the foot. Again, ten seconds slow, ten seconds moderate, and ten seconds as fast as possible.
3.   **Tire jumping.** Back and forth. You don't need actual tires for this. Fifteen seconds moderate, fifteen seconds fast.
4.   **Shallow jumping lunges. Knee does not go past the toe** unless you hate your body and want it to break down. Start with your feet together and take a step forward with your right leg. Your left leg should be stretched back so your left knee is bent and the left foot stands on the toes. Right leg is a bit higher than parallel to the floor. Keep your core tight and shoulders back. Push off the right heel, jump, switch the legs in mid-air, repeat. Fifteen seconds moderate, fifteen seconds fast.
5.   **Lunges.** Same as before, but deeper, with the right thigh getting parallel to the floor at the deepest moment, and no jumping. Just stand up, legs together, switch legs, repeat. Do it at a calm pace for a minute and a half.
6.   **Deep prayer squats.** Start with your feet wider than yours shoulders at approximately 45 degree angle. Raise your hands up vertically; bend down so your torso makes a 45 degree angle with the floor. Move your arms perpendicular to the torso; bend down by pushing the hips back so your arms touch your inner feet. Hips down as low as you can, and put your arms in the "praying" position, pushing your knees out with your elbows. Hold for a

second, then raise the arms up, and squat up. Repeat 30 times at a calm pace.

That's it, you've done the warm-up. As your performance increases and you feel more confident, feel free to go hard, starting from step 3. And if you enjoy doing the exercises described here, you can make the warm-up a full-fledged cardio workout by doing it several times in a row.

Stretching

Stretching is great. It protects you from injury, increases your performance, makes you more flexible, and is just plain pleasant to do. If it hurts and is uncomfortable, you're doing something wrong. One big tip here is to breathe. Breathe in deeply, then relax and go a bit deeper into stretch as you breathe out.

1. **Standing quad stretch**. Find something for support if keeping balance standing on one leg is hard for you. Grab your ankle and pull your heel up and back. Gently pull until you feel a stretch in your thigh. Keep your knees together, and tighten your core. Hold for thirty seconds, then change legs and repeat.

2. **Hamstring stretch.** Lie down on your back, legs straight, arms on your stomach. Raise your right leg up perpendicular to the floor while keeping the right knee bent. Grab your right leg with both arms and straighten out the knee gradually until you start feeling a stretch in your left back thigh. Hold for thirty seconds, and switch legs.

3. **Calf stretch.** Position yourself an arm's length from a wall, and place your right foot back. Bend your left leg forward while making sure your right leg is straight, and right heel is on the floor. If you have problems keeping the heel on the floor, try to lift the toes of your right foot up. You should feel a stretch in your right calf. Hold for thirty seconds, switch legs.

4. **Knee-to-chest stretch.** Lie down on your back, legs straight. Grab your left leg by the upper shin just below the

elbow and bring the left knee to your chest until you feel a stretch in your lower back. Hold for thirty seconds, switch legs.

5. **Shoulder stretch.** Stand up with your legs shoulder width apart. Position your straight right arm across your chest perpendicular to the floor, and press on it gently with the forearm of your left arm. Hold the position for thirty seconds, switch arms.

The stretching is finished, and you can get to the rest of the workout. Pick one that's appropriate, and remember to go hard, but keep control over your movements and maintain proper form.

Quick and Dirty Yoga

If you have time, it pays to do a bit of yoga after a workout, too. Sun Salutation is great, as it isn't complicated, doesn't take much time, and benefits your flexibility, balance, coordination, strength, and endurance. And you aren't tied to a work out. You can do Sun Salutation sequence at any time of the day, coupled with a workout or by itself. It isn't effective at pumping up your muscles or burning off fat, but it's very good for overall health and fitness, and you can do it on off-days, too!

The Workout

Have you heard about High Intensity Interval Training? It's the relatively new big thing in the world of fitness, and one of the best solutions for anyone looking to gain speed and endurance or lose fat. Relatively, because it's been developed back in 1970s and was used by many professional athletes such as Olympic speed skaters, but is only now becoming mainstream. It's very efficient at burning off fat and increasing endurance, but unlike conventional cardio it's much less time consuming, and it also gives strength, speed, and agility benefits. There are several variants of High Intensity Interval Training (HIIT).

Gibala regimen. This HIIT regimen is the easier one. Beginner and intermediate athletes alike should utilize it. It involves several minutes of warm-up followed by 60 seconds of intense exercise followed by 75 seconds of rest, repeated for several cycles. It's what beginner and intermediate cardio plyo workouts were developed around. Imagine you are a ninja jogging silently through the woods. That's the rest and warm-up stages. Now imagine you are a ninja being chased by a bear. That's how much you should push yourself during an intense phase. And since you're a ninja, you still have to be silent and control your movements, so you minimize impact and don't end up damaging your joints.

Tabata regimen. More effective, but more hardcore, too. Tabata regimen utilizes 20 seconds of ultra-intense exercise followed by 10 seconds of rest, which is repeated for just 4 minutes. Then you change to another group of exercise, and do another 4 minute cycle. You shouldn't use this regimen unless you're advanced, as you won't be able to push yourself as needed, and won't get its full benefits, Gibala regimen being more effective for you. Remember the bear analogy? Imagine you're a ninja being chased by velociraptors who shoot lasers from their eyes. This is how much you have to push yourself on a Tabata regimen.

On to the workouts. Some general tips:

- Wear cushioned sneakers
- Land as silently as possible to minimize impact
- Don't forget to do the warm-up and stretching. If you skip straight to the workout, say goodbye to your favorite body parts.
- When you contract your muscles when standing up from the squat or lunge, jumping up, or performing a similar movement, exhale sharply and quickly and explode up. When you relax your muscles, going into a squat or lunge, inhale. That way you can keep your breath and exert addition force when contracting the muscles.
- Keep your core tight during all exercise. This will let you generate more power.

Beginner routine

Intense phase:

1. **Squats**. Position your feet a bit wider than shoulder width apart parallel to each other. Squat down until thighs are parallel to the floor while allowing hips to bend back behind. Return to the starting position. Remember to keep your back straight and torso as upright as possible. Knees must point in the same direction as your feet. You can go lower than parallel with your squat provided you don't feel any discomfort doing it. Contrary to popular belief it won't damage your knees. Do as many as you can as fast as you can for twenty seconds.

2. **Standing jumps.** Squat halfway to parallel and then quickly jump up as high as possible. Clap both hands above your head while jumping. Land into a halfway squat and jump again immediately. Do as many as you can as fast and as high as you can for twenty seconds.

3. **Lunges. Knee does not go past the toe** unless you hate your body and want it to break down. Start with your feet together and take a step forward with your right leg. Your left leg should be stretched back so your left knee is bent and the left foot stands on the toes, while the right thigh is parallel to the floor. Stand up, legs together, step forward with left leg, repeat. Keep your core tight and shoulders back. Do it as fast as possible for twenty seconds.

Resting phase:

1. **Walk briskly or jog in place.** You don't have to go fast during the rest phase, just don't stop. The rest phase lasts for one minute.

Do 10 cycles of intense-resting phases.

After the last resting phase, walk or jog in place for three minutes, gradually slowing down.

Intermediate routine

Intense phase 1:

1. **Suicide drills**. Place two small objects on the floor. They should be at least 6 feet apart from each other. Start by standing near one object, and sprint to the second one. Plant, rush to the other object. Strive to go as fast as you can. **20 seconds.**
2. **Jump lunges.** Start with your feet together and take a step forward with your right leg. Your left leg should be stretched back so your left knee is bent and the left foot stands on the toes. Keep your core tight and shoulders back. Push off the right heel, jump, switch the legs in mid-air, repeat. **20 seconds.**
3. **Mountain climbers.** A standard mountain climber looks is this: position your hands on the floor a bit wider than shoulder width apart. Bend one leg and position it so your knee is close to your chest, and the other leg is extended back. Quickly push up hips and switch legs while the upper body keeps the same position. Remember to contract your core in addition to using your legs. There are several variations. Feel free to use any of them. **20 seconds.**

Resting phase 1: Jog in place. 60 seconds.

Do 6 cycles of intense-resting phases. When done, move on to Intense phase 2 and rest phase 2.

Intense phase 2:

1. **Jump squats.** Get down into squat position. Go as low as you can. From this position, explode up as high as you can, clap your outstretched arms, land into a low squat, and jump again. **20 seconds.**
2. **Ski jumps.** Stand with your feet shoulder width apart. Bend your knees and go into a half-squat position while maintaining a straight spine. Jump to the left, pushing

off with both feet equally. Softly land into a half-squat position and immediately jump to the right. Repeat. **20 seconds.**

3. **Mountain climbers.** Do a variation different from what you did during phase 1. **20 seconds.**

Resting phase 2: March in place. 60 seconds.

Do 6 cycles of intense-resting phases.

Cool down with five minutes of jogging in place, gradually slowing down.

Advanced routine

This routine is hard. A Tabata protocol performed at proper intensity can burn as much as 13.5 kcal per minute and additional 150kcals afterwards. If you perform it at peak effort, you might not even finish it. Consult a medical specialist. Don't try to continue if you start to feel dizzy.

This is not meant to be performed every day; if you're bent on doing a HIIT routine every day, use the same exercises with a Gibala regimen. As Prof. Tabata said, "If you are doing Tabata correctly (and many people do not) you would only be able to ever do one round of it—and indeed you'd be unlikely to even finish that before complete exhaustion set in! ".

1. **Jump lunges** Start with your feet together and take a step forward with your right leg. Your left leg should be stretched back so your left knee is bent and the left foot stands on the toes. Keep your core tight and shoulders back. Push off the right heel, jump, switch the legs in mid-air, repeat. **20 seconds of going at your absolute max speed. Do as many lunges as you can and then do five more.**

2. **Jog in place for 10 seconds.**

3. **Jump squats.** Get down into squat position. Go as low as you can. From this position, explode up as high as

you can, clap your outstretched arms, land into a low squat, and jump again. **20 seconds of going at your absolute max speed. Do as many squats as fast as you can and then do five more.**

4. **Jog in place for 10 seconds.**
5. **Burpees.** Squat down, place hands on the floor slightly wider than shoulder width, and kick legs back. Do a push-up, and once you've finished, contract the abs and pull legs forward so your feet are touching your palms. Jump up and as you land, go down into the squat position and repeat the exercise. **20 seconds of going at your absolute max speed. Do as many burpees as fast as you can and then do five more.** If you can't do the pushups, return the legs back after you kick them back and go into the squat, then jump, rinse and repeat.
6. **Jog in place for 10 seconds.**
7. **Mountain climbers.** A standard mountain climber looks like this: position your hands on the floor a bit wider than shoulder width apart. Bend one leg and position it so your knee is close to your chest, and the other leg is extended back. Quickly push up hips and switch legs while the upper body keeps the same position. Remember to contract your core in addition to using your legs. There are several variations. Feel free to use any of them. **20 seconds.**
8. **Rest or jog in place for 2 minutes.** Don't stand still, as going from full throttle to stop is bad for your heart.

   If you have the energy left (then you may not be going hard enough)**, repeat the cycle 4 times. Cool down by jogging in place for 5 minutes after the last cycle.**

That's it. You are done! How much calories you burn during this is largely a question of how hard you are going. Here's a tip. If you are doing it every day, consider it heavy exercise; if you are doing it every other day, then it's moderate.

Mind Games

Finally, the neglected part. Psychology is a large part of diet. After all, if you are not committed to the weight loss, you will fail. How to commit, though? We are led to believe that you have to bust through your cravings with sheer power of will. We are taught that there is no magical pill that will make us not want to eat. Well, guess what? There is a pill. And it works.

There are several mental reasons people fail to lose weight for good.

First reason: people go hard for a week or two, and then burn out. They lose several lbs. of weight while inflicting unimaginable torture upon themselves only to give up later. They aren't weak. The kind of effort that they try to apply is simply unsustainable.

Second reason: people mistake cravings for hunger. People consider stuff like cakes, candies, soda and ice cream tasty. In reality, it's not. It just triggers a response that makes us want more simply because such foods are so, so high in calories. Oh, and also – our bodies don't know when to stop eating. We are always hungry, unless we are literally about to burst.

Third reason: people miscalculate the amount of food they actually consume. There are several reasons behind this, but the biggest and most unexpected one is the size of plates, packs, packets, and packages. They have a major influence on how much we eat, and cause most people mistake the actual number of calories they get a day.

We've identified the psychological problems that don't let people lose weight effectively. What are the solutions?

Solution to problem #1.

Don't go all out. Weight loss is a gradual process. You have nowhere to hurry, unless you are losing weight for a specific event that will happen in a few days. If that's the case, the only advice is to shift to protein and fat, don't eat carbohydrates in the days before the event. The day before the event, minimize intake of liquids. This should make you lose water weight and empty your muscle glycogen stores, resulting in the overall lower size. This is not healthy, and this is not recommended. The weight is just going to come back.

Instead of cutting out all unhealthy foods and going on a caloric deficit AND an exercise routine, do everything gradually.

Start out by limiting your junk food intake. Don't cut it all out. Instead, tell yourself you are only going to try *new* junk foods. If you already had some Oreos, well, that's it. No more Oreos. That bag of chips is still game, though. Eventually you are going to exhaust your options while refusing your comfort foods and you start to not have cravings for junk foods. You'll also realize you were craving not taste, but specific foods that were associated with comfort, reward, or other pleasant things in your mind.

While you are there, take one of your meals and make it healthy. By now you know which foods you should use. Make one meal of your day healthy, for instance that at breakfast, and gradually expand your recipe library. Take your time. There's no need to go from one healthy meal to all three in a day. Your comfort is important here. Do it, and when you are used to it, add dinner to the "healthy meal" list. And if you are not feeling it at this one particular breakfast, you can skip the healthy option and put it in place of supper, for instance.

Do the same thing for calories. Don't go for a 500kcal deficit at once. Instead, use portions that are a bit smaller in high GI, high GL food department, but higher in vegetables and protein. If you are making spaghetti with tomatoes, decrease the amount of spaghetti while increasing the amount of tomatoes. Gradually increase the proportion of tomatoes until you are where you want to be.

Solution to problem #2

Ah, cravings. The bane of every dieter. And something that is very easy to get rid of using proper psychological tools. After all, denying yourself the pleasures of life is bad, right? Right.

So here's what you are going to do. First, remember the rule of "always new"? If you can reliably classify something as a junk food, you can only have it once. After that, move on to the next junk food. Oh, and here's one more rule: if you don't like it, you still have to eat it all before you try new junk food. Seems easy, right? That's because it is.

The other thing to do to get rid of cravings is to make getting that fix a bit harder. Don't place the bowl of candy close to you. Place it far enough you actually have to get up and walk to it. Put it somewhere you don't see it all the time. The darker, unexplored regions of cupboards are a great place for candy. And when you want to buy some, just remember you have a jar of it at home, waiting for you in that cupboard.

Spend time reading the labels, too. Read not only the macronutrient break-up of your junk food of choice. Read all the ingredients. Remember that if it's at the start of the list then it's the chief ingredient. Now imagine how it looks at the manufacturing plant. All those vats of oil and sugar. Why not go one step further when visualizing this thing? If you are buying your junk food to eat at home, read the list of ingredients and put an appropriate amount of sugar and oil on top of that particular representative of junk food. If for instance you've bought "Dirty Eating Habits" chocolate bar with 30g sugar and 30g oil (yep, oil is used in cheap chocolate bars; if it's actually real cocoa fat, it's good for you), put it in your fridge, and place two little cups containing 30g sugar and 30g oil on top of it. This is just to help you better realize what you eat. Or just put a cup containing the caloric value of your junk food in oil. This oil is going to end up as your body fat.

Finally, if you have a sweet tooth, go for dark. Dark chocolate is actually good for you, and while it still has a high GI and GL – a thing to avoid – the benefits outweigh the drawbacks, at least if you don't care about losing weight. If you do care, just make sure it fits in your daily caloric intake.

Solution to problem #3

The leading causes behind obesity are cravings and inability to control portion size. We've dealt with cravings. Now, on to portion size. This is even easier. There are three rules here. Container size, memento rule and apple rule.

> **Container size.** This goes for jars, cans, sacks, plates, cups, mugs. Everything you use to store food should be small. If you buy a large back of chips, place them in small bowls. The smaller, the better. Don't say "I am going to eat less chips" and fight yourself for the next few hours until you give up. Instead, distribute the large bag of chips between several smaller plastic containers, and then fill up a small bowl or plate with chips. Make the bowl small, but fill it to the edge. Same with goes for everything else. Use smaller glasses, plates, pans for cooking and eating. Use smaller dishes, but fill them up.

> **Something to remember food by, or the memento rule.** As we already said, human bodies are bad at measuring satiety and the amount of food they consumed. The only reminder of how much you ate are the leftovers. Leave wrapping lying around until you decide you are not having any more of those candies, because as soon as you throw the wrappings away, your unconscious candy counter will be back to 0, and you'll start eating the candy again.

> **Apple rule.** This rule was devised to combat both cravings and inability to control portions. It's actually very simple. Are you feeling hungry? Yes? Would you like an apple? If you answer "no", then it's cravings. Apples, while being tasty, are low in things that our bodies crave. Namely, fats and sugars. Not many people crave apples, and if they do, the apples don't cause obesity, being low in calories and low in GL. So go on – ask yourself. "Do I feel like I want an apple? Do I?"
> And if you do, by all means, have one.

Observe these principles, and you will find yourself leaner and healthier than you were in no time, while your cravings will be gone.

The trick isn't to push and punish yourself.

The trick is to reach your goal. And in dieting like nowhere else slow and steady wins the race.

So go on – start slow.

Squat down until thighs are parallel to the floor while allowing hips to bend back behind. Return to the starting position. Remember to keep your back straight and torso as upright as possible. Knees must point in the same direction as your feet. You can go lower than parallel with your squat provided you don't feel any discomfort doing it.

ABOUT THE AUTHOR

Charles Thornton RN BSN is an expert in exercise and weight loss.

Determined to help others prevent heart disease.

Other Books by the author

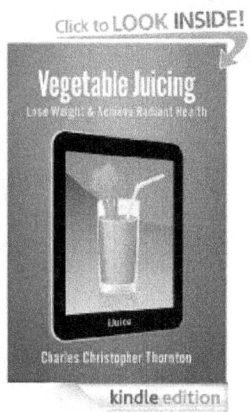

Click to LOOK INSIDE!

Click to open expanded view

Share your own customer images

Vegetable Juicing: Lose Weight & Achieve Radiant Health [Kindle Edition]

Charles Christopher Thornton (Author)
Be the first to review this item

Digital List Price: ~~$9.99~~ What's this? ☑

Kindle Price: **$8.49**

You Save: $1.50 (15%)

Length: 112 pages (estimated) ☑

Don't have a Kindle? Get your Kindle here.

Whispersync for Voice: Ready ☑

Whispersync for Voice

Now you can switch back and forth between reading the Kindle book and listening to the Audible audiobook. Learn more

Add the professional narration of Vegetable Juicing: Lose Weight & Achieve Radiant Health **for a reduced price of** $1.99 after you buy this Kindle book.

Formats	Amazon Price	New from	Used from
Kindle Edition	$8.49	--	--
Audible Audio Edition, Unabridged	$10.46 or 1 credit		

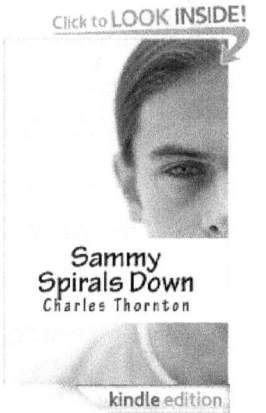

Click to LOOK INSIDE!

Sammy Spirals Down
Charles Thornton

kindle edition

Click to open expanded view

Share your own customer images

Sammy Spirals Down [Kindle Edition]

Charles Thornton (Author)

Be the first to review this item

Print List Price: ~~$5.99~~

Kindle Price: $2.99

You Save: $3.00 (50%)

Length: **96 pages** ⌄

Don't have a Kindle? Get your Kindle here.

Whispersync for Voice: Ready ⌄

Whispersync for Voice

Now you can switch back and forth between reading the Kindle book and listening to the Audible audiobook. Learn more

Add the professional narration of Sammy Spirals Down **for a reduced price of** $1.99 after you buy this Kindle book.

Formats	Amazon Price	New from	Used from
Kindle Edition	$2.99	--	--
Expand Paperback	$5.69	$5.69	--
Audible Audio Edition, Unabridged	$10.46 or 1 credit		

Share

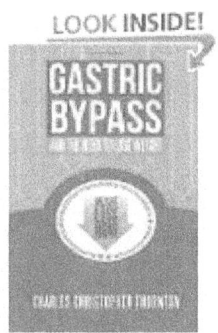

Gastric Bypass and the Need to Lose Weight by Charles Christopher Thornton (Jun 12, 2013)

Formats	Price	New	Used

PaperbackIn stock but may require an extra 1-2 days to process. FREE Shipping on orders over $35

~~$20.49~~ **$18.44**

Kindle Edition Auto-delivered wirelessly

$0.00 (read for free, Join Amazon Prime)
$2.99 to buy

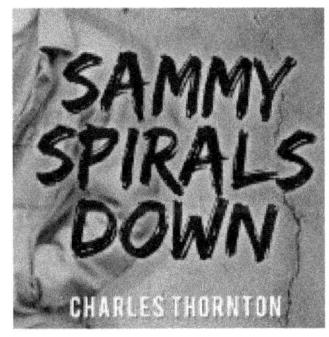

[Sammy Spirals Down](#) by Charles Christopher Thornton and Mimi Spillane (Jun 2, 2013) - **Unabridged**

Formats	Price	New	Used
Audible Audio Edition Whispersync for Voice-ready	**$13.08**		
Kindle Edition Whispersync for Voice-ready	**$2.99**		

Other Formats: Paperback

Thanks for your purchase